Distribution, publication, and copying in any form are prohibited and subject to damages.

TEN HYPNOSES

Copying, publishing, and sharing with third parties are only permitted with the written consent of the author. Please observe the notes on copyright and usage.

Distribution, publication, and copying in any form are prohibited and subject to damages.

Copying, publishing, and sharing with third parties are only permitted with the written consent of the author. Please observe the notes on copyright and usage.

Distribution, publication, and copying in any form are prohibited and subject to damages.

Ingo Michael Simon

TEN HYPNOSES

13

Depressive Thoughts

Copying, publishing, and sharing with third parties are only permitted with the written consent of the author. Please observe the notes on copyright and usage.

Distribution, publication, and copying in any form are prohibited and subject to damages.

© 2024 Ingo Michael Simon
All rights reserved.
Independently published
www.ingosimon.com

Important Notes for Urgent Attention:
The contents of this book are based on the practical experiences of the author with hypnosis applications and psychotherapy in a trance state. Although the author has strived for the utmost care, errors or misunderstandings in the presentation cannot be completely excluded. Therapeutic work with people and the application of hypnosis are solely the responsibility of the hypnotist. It cannot be ruled out that parts of this book may be misunderstood or that the application of a presented procedure may cause an undesirable reaction in the client. The author also assumes no co-responsibility if work with a client is carried out with reference to the statements in this book.

The Author:
Ingo Michael Simon studied psychology and education and is a hypnotherapist with practices in southwestern Germany and Switzerland. With the help of hypnosis-supported psychotherapy, he primarily treats people with persistent psychological conditions. His practice focuses on anxiety disorders, pathological compulsions, and psychosomatic illnesses. His therapeutic offerings mainly include classical and modern hypnosis applications and the dreamland therapy he developed himself.

Copying, publishing, and sharing with third parties are only permitted with the written consent of the author. Please observe the notes on copyright and usage.

Distribution, publication, and copying in any form are prohibited and subject to damages.

Notes on Copyright and Usage

Copying, publishing, and sharing with third parties is prohibited and only permitted with the written consent of the author. Please observe the following copyright and usage guidelines.

This work has been carefully crafted and created to the best of the author's knowledge and personal experience. It comprises text templates and application guidelines for professional hypnosis sessions. The author is a licensed psychotherapist with extensive experience in psychotherapy, coaching, and personal training using hypnotic techniques and methods. Nevertheless, the author and the publisher assume no liability for the accuracy of information, instructions, and advice, nor for any typographical errors. The author and publisher accept no responsibility or liability for the application of these texts and recommendations with clients or patients, nor for any potential consequences or unexpected reactions. It is expressly noted that the application of therapeutic and advisory techniques and formulations lies solely and entirely within the responsibility of the practitioner. This also applies to adherence to the boundaries of legally regulated medical and therapeutic practices. The fact that a book containing action proposals is freely available for sale does not imply that its application with clients or patients is permitted for everyone.

Copying, publishing, and sharing with third parties are only permitted with the written consent of the author. Please observe the notes on copyright and usage.

Distribution, publication, and copying in any form are prohibited and subject to damages.

Copying, publishing, and sharing with third parties are only permitted with the written consent of the author. Please observe the notes on copyright and usage.

Distribution, publication, and copying in any form are prohibited and subject to damages.

Table of Contents

Introduction 9

#1 11

#2 16

#3 20

#4 26

#5 32

#6 37

#7 42

#8 47

#9 52

#10 57

Overview of All Titles in the Series "Ten Hypnoses" 62

Copying, publishing, and sharing with third parties are only permitted with the written consent of the author. Please observe the notes on copyright and usage.

Distribution, publication, and copying in any form are prohibited and subject to damages.

Copying, publishing, and sharing with third parties are only permitted with the written consent of the author. Please observe the notes on copyright and usage.

Introduction

The series "Ten Hypnoses" is very well known in Germany, Austria, and Switzerland as a collection of texts for therapeutic work and is used by numerous psychotherapeutic practices, doctors, therapists, coaches, and other helping professionals. I am pleased to now be able to offer these texts in other countries as well.

Most therapists have their own methods for inducing and deepening trance as well as for exiting trance. Therefore, I have focused on the main part of the hypnosis. The texts in this book can be integrated as the main part into any hypnosis process.

The texts in this collection use various hypnosis techniques. I will not explain these in detail, as I assume that users have the appropriate training. It is also not necessary to understand the exact structure or functioning of the different parts. The texts can simply be read aloud, and they will have their effect.

Decide for yourself which text best suits your client or patient at any given time. You can also combine passages from different texts. It is not about using all ten hypnoses in sequence. It is a selection of possibilities.

I want to emphasize that books cannot replace therapy. Psychotherapy or other therapeutic treatments involve much more. A careful diagnosis is the necessary basis for deciding on the use of methods, including whether hypnosis or one of my texts should be used. Even in this case, preparatory discussions, follow-up discussions during the session, and of course, a therapeutic concept for the sequence of sessions and the content approaches are essential parts of therapy. This cannot and should not be achieved with a collection of texts.

In any case, I wish you much success in your work and I am pleased if my text templates can contribute in a small way.

Ingo Michael Simon

#1

You want to let go of your heavy thoughts to finally become light again ... ... to feel light inside ... ... Maybe you think it can't be so easy to be completely free again ... ... but perhaps it is easier than you think ... ... Many things can be easier when we allow ourselves to embrace them ... ... and you have decided to embark on a new path now ... ... a path deep into trance ... ... because in the depths of relaxation, everything is lighter ... ... much lighter ... ... You don't have to do or achieve anything now ... ... It is enough to simply be here and find peace ... ... in fact, you have already found it, because you have become calmer inside ... ... So you have already taken an important step toward relief ... ... But there is more to come ... ... Today you can find deep inner peace ... ... a very deep inner peace ... ... Peace means relief, because thoughts that burdened you in a waking state are now much smaller and lighter ... ... Truly remarkable how well you are managing to go even deeper into trance now ... ... even deeper into inner relaxation and peace ... ... It becomes easier for you with every breath … … with every single breath, you relax deeper and deeper … …

… … Some people feel heavier in relaxation because their bodies relax the muscles … … If that's the case for you, it just shows that you are becoming lighter inside … … because a heavy body indicates relaxation … … and relaxation means lightness in mood … … lightness in your thoughts … … lightness in your feelings … … Perhaps your body feels lighter too, because many people experience a feeling of floating and freedom in trance … … maybe it's the same for you … … But deep inside, deep in your feelings, everything is light … … You can feel it if you focus on your center … … on your gut feeling … … It becomes lighter inside you … … much lighter … …

… … You can also imagine that all the thoughts that were so heavy are slowly flowing away … … flowing away with every exhale … … The more you focus on the feeling of exhaling, the faster and easier you can feel the heavy thoughts leaving … … So, feel your breath consciously and follow the movement of your body … … Exhaling feels light … … Exhaling feels liberating … … Breathe out and feel free … … good … … very good … … Truly amazing how easily you manage to become lighter … … lighter and lighter … … So, you feel a sense of freedom rising within you again … … remembering how it was in the past when you felt much lighter anyway … … The memory of a carefree, free time rises within you, along with the feeling of freedom and inner lightness … … Now you can rest and just be, that is enough … … In this peace, new strength arises within you … … a hint of cheerfulness … … and with every breath, with every hint of your breath, the idea of cheerfulness becomes more intense … … You want to be cheerful again … … to be cheerful and stay cheerful … … and your deep inner self is fully aligned to make that possible … … to be cheerful and stay cheerful … … You start today … … and it happens effortlessly … … You don't have to do or achieve anything … … You want to experience joy again, and with that, you have made a decision … … Now, in the state of trance, a simple decision becomes truth in your feeling … … truly amazing how quickly your organism implements this decision for you … … Perhaps you have already noticed that your body has adopted a different posture as a sign of change … … maybe you will feel it a little later … … The relaxation of your body shows the inner lightness and freedom that have already arisen and are growing with every breath ... ... and your body shows this relaxation ... ... It has adopted a noticeably more relaxed posture ... ... Perhaps you notice it yourself now if you pay attention to your body feeling ... ... if you now feel into your body and realize that you can actually feel a noticeable relaxation ... ... Maybe all this doesn't matter so much ... ... maybe you just want to enjoy being here and having your peace ... ... then you feel the calm mood ... ... the inner relaxation ... ... Wherever you feel the peace and relaxation, it is indeed within you and spreading ... ... whether first in your body, whose relaxation and lightness you can feel ... ... or first in your inner feeling, in the mood, whose relaxation and lightness you can feel ... ... Everything is light inside you ... ... everything is light ... ... Truly remarkable how well you are managing to let all this arise inside you just as you hear it from me ... ... Truly amazing how well you have already let go of all burdens and how quickly you are letting them go ... ... So, you allow yourself complete peace, because you have already accomplished and achieved a lot ... ... Maybe you have felt that you are the one making all this possible ... ... Maybe you have noticed that you can bring about any change within yourself with your own thoughts ... ... But perhaps you didn't notice it and just felt that it feels better inside you ... ... Then you now think about how it always becomes easier for you to let go of all burdens and feel light again ... ... to repeatedly enter a state of letting go and inner lightness ... ... just like today ... ... exactly like today ... ...

What you have achieved today, you achieve every day ... ... Everything you have reached today, you can reach every day ... ... Today's peace can arise every day ... ... Today's lightness can arise every day and become even more intense ... ... You tell yourself every day when you wake up in the morning ... ... Yes, I can be light and cheerful again today ... ... This sentence accompanies you and becomes your new creed ... ... Yes, I can be light and cheerful again today ... ... and whenever you want to come into a lighter feeling and a better, more cheerful mood, you say it again ... ... Yes, I can be light and cheerful again today ... ... This is how you succeed every day ... ... just like today ... ... exactly like today ... ...

#2

You have a deep desire to finally let go of the circling thoughts and find a pleasant peace and inner silence as quickly as possible ... ... You are fully committed to achieving this goal as soon as possible ... ... You are particularly successful in focusing on this one thought and letting your thoughts revolve around this single wish ... ... Quieting thoughts ... ... deep, inner quieting thoughts ... ... For so long, the same thoughts have been bothering and weakening you ... ... but today you are turning things around ... ... Today you can use the circling thoughts for yourself ... ... to finally become free again ... ... So you decide that your thoughts will revolve around this one wish ... ... Circling and recurring thoughts can be very persistent ... ... You know this because you have already had this experience ... ... But sometimes a persistent thought can also be helpful ... ... a thought that is constructive and leads to a real breakthrough ... ... and your thought about quieting thoughts is exactly such a persistent thought ... ... your will is stable and firm ... ... You want to experience peace and inner silence ... ... You want it, and that is why your thoughts are now set on it ... ... Even if other persistent thoughts cling to you and follow you, your thought about quieting thoughts is always there ... ... Your desire for peace and inner silence clings to all other thoughts ... ... Truly amazing how well you manage to make the circling thoughts something really helpful ... ... Fantastic how you do it, that just the brooding helps you become free ... ... You have found a way to now use the repetition of thoughts constructively, because you repeat the thought of finally becoming free ... ... finding inner peace ... ... Only this one thought circles, and only this one thought comes to the forefront ... ... Quieting thoughts ... ... Quieting thoughts ... ... You are doing it right ... ... You prescribe the thinking to yourself ... ... the thinking about liberation and inner peace ... ... You actually manage to prescribe this to your organism ... ... For a long time, you have suffered from constantly circling thoughts and always tried to let them go or end them ... ... Now you simply do it differently ... ... You use the constant thoughts to establish exactly this one thought ... ... the thought of silence ... ... the thought of peace ... ... the thought of quieting thoughts ... ...

… … [Now follows a sequence of guided breathing. Make sure to speak the following suggestions for inhaling and exhaling in the rhythm of the client's actual breathing. However, stretch the suggestion "breathe out slowly and long" a bit to slow down the breathing. This happens automatically if you first speak exactly in the client's rhythm and then become a bit slower.] … …

… … Now focus entirely on your breathing … … Now it is only about your breathing … … Take a deep breath in and slowly and long out [Stretch] … … good, and again … … deep breath in and slowly and long out [Stretch] … … deep breath in … … and slowly and long out [Stretch] … … in … … and out [Stretch] … … in … … and out [Stretch] … … Good, very good … … in … … and out [Stretch] … … and now allow yourself peace and relaxation … … Just keep breathing in your own rhythm … … in your tempo, at your own speed … …

… … That's right … … Perhaps you noticed that while focusing on your breathing, you couldn't think of anything else but breathing … … The other thoughts had no room … … it has almost become quieter … … much quieter … … This one important thought about inner silence is already working

... ... It is already working deep within you because now you could follow a completely different thought ... ... the simple thought about the rhythm of your breathing ... ... You have just experienced how easy it is to stop circling thoughts if you just manage to hold onto a new and different thought ... ... for example, the thought about your breathing ... ... But you have managed to make a very special thought work, even and especially when you no longer pay attention to it ... ... because this special thought is indeed always there ... ... the thought about quieting thoughts ... ... You have made it so strong and so effective ... ... You feel that it works ... ... even more, you have experienced that it works ... ... So you have already managed to interrupt circling thoughts ... ... You have managed it here and today ... ... and so you will manage it again every day ... ...

Your organism memorizes this exactly. It knows that the special thought about silence always works for you ... ... even and especially when you no longer observe the thoughts and simply let them go ... ... So you prescribe yourself a time of conscious breathing every day ... ... You lie down and close your eyes and just observe your breathing ... ... follow each breath ... ... and at the same time, this one thought, which continues on and on … … the thought of peace and quiet within you … … Peace and quiet within you … … just like today … … exactly like today … … Peace and quiet within you … …

#3

The following variant of a hypnosis main part works with an anchor in the form of a handy card with a printed sun symbol. This can simply be a drawn sun, i.e., a golden-yellow circle with a few "rays." An anchor is a trigger that should create a specific feeling or evoke a particular thought. We want to help the client use a symbol card to brighten their mood when they notice that their mood is declining. Discuss this with the client before the session and prepare the symbol card. It can be a blank business card or similar. Simply draw a simple sun on it. The card is prepared and given to the client to hold during hypnosis or place on their body, preferably on the solar plexus. They should carry the card with them after the hypnosis session, in their pants or jacket pocket.

You have the goal of finally consigning the bad mood to the past ... ... placing it in the realm of memory and leaving it there ... ... because that is where depression belongs ... ... You are now setting yourself up for lightness ... ... You can recall the events and experiences of the depressive period in your memory, but they should not enter the present ... ... because the present belongs only to you ... ... The time of clinging to old thought patterns and depression is now over ... ... It is important that we hold on just as long as we need to process and understand what has happened ... ... You have now reached this point ... ... You have processed and understood ... ... Therefore, now is the right time to let go ... ... to let go of the feelings of the past and thus the feelings of depression ... ...

... ... You have decided that you want to let go ... ... You have understood that you can thus make room for new and pleasant feelings ... ... You know that it is you who makes your success ... ... and you are ready for it ... ... You are ready to give everything necessary to become internally free ... ... free from old heavy thoughts ... ... You have the potential ... ... you have the strength you need ... ... You think of the warmth of a beautiful sun ... ... Lying in the sun and sleeping gives a warm and healing feeling ... ... and today it can be the same ... ... Today a sun inside you can make your mood shine ... ... because the power of the sun dissolves the old thought patterns and brightens the mood ... ... Sun inside you ... ... Sun inside you ... ...

... ... You have this card with the sun symbol in your hand ... ... Sun brightens the mood ... ... This phrase, together with the sun symbol card, becomes your new belief ... ... your new inner truth ... ... You feel now this inner power that is growing more and more within you ... ... You know that you can accomplish anything ... ... your will and your willingness are growing with every breath, and with every breath, it becomes clearer ... ... Sun brightens the mood ... ... The card shows it to you every day ... ... It shows you your development path, which you can always carry as a symbol ... ... Sun brightens the mood ... ... The sun symbol helps you to feel better every day and eventually to be free again ... ... Whenever even the slightest doubt arises because you feel your mood slipping, you immediately take the card in your hand and look closely at the sun symbol ... ... Sun brightens the mood ... ... Then you immediately feel the effect, you feel that this is your truth ... ... You do it every day ... ... You simply let go of the depression ... ... You just let go of the past ... ...

The card shows it to you every day ... It shows you your own attitude, which you can always carry with you ... ... It helps you through difficult moments ... ... Whenever even the slightest doubt arises in you or your mood threatens to slip, you immediately take the card in your hand and look at it ... ... Sun brightens the mood ... ... Then you immediately feel the effect, you feel that this is your truth ... ...

... ... Now take your symbol card very consciously in your hand ... ... Hold it tightly ... ... Have you noticed that you are holding onto something again? ... ... This time you are holding onto the sun ... ... and as unbelievable and paradoxical as it may sound ... ... That is a good holding on ... ... holding on to your goal of being happy and free again ... ... holding on to the fact that you are important to yourself ... ... holding on to your goal of freeing yourself ... ... holding on to the fact that there is nothing more important to you than finally letting go of the depression ... ... holding on only to the moment of the present ... ... holding on only to the moment of the present ... ... Already in the next second, the present is over ... ... and everything that is over, you let go ... ... The card that you feel between your fingers reminds you of this ... ... it helps you let go of the heavy thoughts and thus brighten your mood … … Sun brightens the mood … … it helps you to be free and to take new paths … … to go freely and openly towards the future … … freely and openly … … every day … … Place the card on your body … … right on your solar plexus, because that is where the sun belongs … … Place the card on your solar plexus and feel the warmth and healing power of the sun … … good, you are doing it right … … This way, the sun's power works deeply within you and brightens your mood … … The more you focus on your solar plexus, the better you feel the effect … … feel that your mood is indeed brightening … …

… … [Now instruct the client to open their eyes and look at the symbol while in trance. This enhances the effect. Opening the eyes is a fractionation, which can be done without special announcement or counting. Everyone can open their eyes in trance. In a stable and deep trance, it is somewhat laborious because the client is tired and sluggish. Just stay suggestive until the eyes are opened and the card is looked at. If you prefer to initiate the fractionation through counting steps, you can do that. It is not necessary, though.] … …

… … Now take the card once again in your hand and feel it very consciously between your fingers, and if you want, open your eyes briefly and look at the card … … open your eyes and look at what you see on it … … You see the sun symbol, which tells you … … Sun brightens the mood … … Now close your eyes again and rest … …

You know that the sun symbol can remind you every day to become free by letting go … … Whenever you take the card in your hand and see the sun symbol, you immediately feel that your mood brightens … … Whenever you carry the card with you, you quickly get into a good mood … … Sun brightens the mood … … Sun brightens the mood … …

#4

Agitated Depression

The following hypnosis session works with a physical anchor. An anchor is a trigger that should create a specific feeling or evoke a particular thought. We want to help the client produce a feeling of inner calm with a slight pressure on the left hand (on the ball below the thumb). Discuss this with the client before the session and show them the spot they should press. During the hypnosis session, we will establish the anchor. It is crucial that the client is subjectively calm and relaxed during this session. This must be absolutely ensured; otherwise, it will not work.

An agitated depression is a mood disorder that does not manifest in subjectively depressed affectivity but in physical restlessness and agitation. This can be experienced as anxious restlessness but can also be accompanied by a subjective urge for activity and may appear superficially not very depressive. Affected individuals can be quite productive, for example, by engaging in intense sports to channel their restlessness.

You have now realized that the agitation and restlessness within you stem from your mood disorder ... ... You didn't expect that it could be a depression leading to this agitation ... ... Perhaps you thought that a depressive mood always comes with sluggishness and lethargy ... ... But sometimes it is different ... ... Sometimes our mood is weighed down by worries or fears, but we don't perceive it that way ... ... You had this distinct feeling, this urge to move ... ... perhaps to move something, to change something ... ... to somehow get out of it ... ... Now you have understood this restlessness, recognized that there is also fear behind it ... ... maybe fear of loss ... ... or existential fears ... ... You can now better look at and process all of this calmly because you know now that it is depression that led to this agitation ... ... For now, it is important to become calmer to interrupt this inner running and pacing, this up-and-down walking, and to find strength again ... ... Strength to process all the issues and worries ... ...

... ... Today we will work with an anchor, we have already discussed this ... ... This anchor is already on your body ... ... your left hand is the anchor that will be triggered by your right hand ... ... But we will get to that a little later ... ... To use the anchor fully, find the best position to trigger it ... ... Reach with your right hand to your left and feel for the ball of your thumb with your fingers ... ... very gently ... ... very softly ... ... Decide whether you prefer to grip with your thumb and index finger or with your thumb and middle finger ... ... perhaps you have another variant ... ... Do it the way you can best grasp the ball of your thumb ... ... [Wait until the client has found a good grip; encourage again if they do not "participate" immediately] ... ... Wonderful ... ... This works best ... ... very good ... ... And now let go of your hand again and place both hands lightly beside your body ... ...

... ... Now it's time to find a very deep relaxation ... ... deeper than ever before ... ... because in the depths of relaxation, you are calm and composed, you get out of the agitation ... ... You go deeper and deeper into yourself ... ... as if you could sink into yourself ... ... You let go of all thoughts ... ... and you pay close attention to your body feeling ... ... You feel how calm you are at this moment ... ... You are truly composed, have no desire to move ... ... Isn't it remarkable how easily it comes to you to feel this sensation so clearly? ... ... Once you have made a decision, you can act on it ... ... You make it absolutely clear to yourself at this moment that you have already made a decision ... ... You have decided to become calmer and more composed to interrupt the agitation ... ... to take good care of yourself ... ... So you need no more than a single second to act on your decision ... ... You simply do what is necessary to make your decision a reality ... ... to feel that you can be and remain calm ... ... just like now ... ... Now, at this very moment, you can feel that you are truly calm inside ... ... You feel the deep desire within you to feel this sensation again and again whenever even the slightest restlessness could arise ... ... You know how it feels when the restlessness arises, and you suddenly feel the need to do something ... ... to take action ... ... You know how it feels when the urge comes up, the inner agitation ... ... Then you want to take immediate countermeasures to become calmer as quickly as possible ... ... Feel the inner calm now ... ... Feel the composure now ... ... Feel the inner calm more and more clearly ... ... Feel the composure more and more clearly ... ... This is good ... ... You are doing it excellently ... ... You are doing it really excellently ... ...

... ... You have decided, so you can act ... ... Now you can indeed act ... ... Grab your left hand ... ... Do it now as you practiced ... ... Grasp your left hand and focus on your inner feeling of calm ... ... If you think the feeling of calm should become even clearer, then simply let it become even clearer and more vivid in your feeling ... ... Just breathe deeply and slowly and long exhale and relax deeper ... ... even deeper ... ... with even more mindfulness and care for yourself ... ... just like that ... ... just like that ... ... You can do it ... ...

... ... And now let this feeling of calm become very conscious ... ... and now press the ball of your left hand ... ... and again ... ... press ... ... Your inner self sets up that exactly this pressing of the ball of the hand is the signal to immediately feel that you are indeed becoming calmer ... ... Whenever you press the ball of your hand, you feel that you become calmer right away ... ... simultaneously, you feel the desire to be careful with yourself ... ... to take yourself seriously ... ... to be important to yourself ... ... Your body is relaxed, and also your hands are completely calm ... ... Your body has understood how your anchor works ... ... It has already stored it for you so that you can use it again and again ... ...

… … Whenever you press the ball of your hand, you will immediately become calmer … … as calm as now … … and feel the need to be mindful with yourself … … to take yourself seriously … … to be important to yourself … … This will soon become second nature to you, to always press or massage the ball of your hand, it works just the same … … exactly the same as now … … You have decided … … You have acted … …

#5

You are here today to dissolve your depression ... ... Sometimes it feels like your thoughts and feelings are walled in ... ... as solid as a rock and no longer movable ... ... Then you feel exactly like that ... ... you can hardly move and muster up any energy ... ... you feel like a huge stone ... ... like a rock ... ... At the same time, you have the desire to simply dissolve this huge block ... ... You imagine how it would be if the stony thoughts and feelings were a rock that slowly turns to sand ... ... Maybe it's just a picture, just an idea ... ... but maybe it's also more ... ... because inner pictures become feelings and thus truth when we engage with them ... ... So if you can connect the picture of a crumbling rock with your thoughts and feelings, then these too will crumble to sand and dust ... ... Perhaps you are wondering how best to achieve this ... ... I will help you with that ... ... it is easier than you think ... ... You will succeed in your imagination ... ... in your creative fantasy ... ... Let your thoughts wander ... ... let them drift and let pictures arise before your inner eye ... ... Imagine you are outside in nature ... ... in a place that you can really like ... ... perhaps on a meadow ... ... or high in the mountains ... ... perhaps you prefer deep valleys and imagine being in a beautiful valley ... ... or you love the sea and imagine being on a beautiful sandy beach ... ... Do it in a way that suits you best ... ... find your favorite place ... ... It is probably very easy for you to imagine a beautiful place ... ... We create inner pictures all day long ... ... imagining the most beautiful things in our daydreams ... ... So now you imagine a beautiful place ... ... your favorite place ... ... and right in front of you is a thick rock ... ... like a boulder that has been thrown into the beautiful landscape ... ... This stone is to symbolize your gloomy thoughts ... ... as a symbol for your feelings that have made you so immobile and melancholic ... ... also as a symbol for the physical lethargy that has set in ... ... You think again about how this depression, this gloom developed ... ... perhaps slowly over years ... ... maybe you only noticed it when it was already very pronounced and in retrospect, you now see that it had been brewing for a long time ... ... Perhaps it also broke out very suddenly ... ... was just there, and you could no longer react to avert it ... ... Perhaps there have been several phases of depressive moods that have gone very differently ... ... Just look again in your mind at how all this came about ... ... how the mood changed over time ... ... Then imagine that all memories of it and all feelings of depression go into this rock and make it even bigger and more solid ... ... So the heavy boulder in front of you grows ... ... it becomes bigger and firmer ... ... because all your depressive feelings, the sadness and fatigue, the lethargy and lack of drive are in this one thick boulder in front of you ... ... The more you imagine that all depressive feelings and difficulties are in this rock, the more freely you can already breathe ... ... It is as if you have already pushed the depression away from you ... ... But you want more ... ... You want to finally dissolve these gloomy feelings and memories, all these blocking thoughts, to stop carrying this rock with you ... ...

... ... You feel your breath, which in your imagination becomes the wind ... ... a wind blowing across the landscape in which you find yourself in this daydream ... ... With each breath, this wind blows over the rock of depression ... ... and with each gust of wind from your breath, some stone crumbles from the rock ... ... You just have to imagine it vividly ... ... The more clearly you can see this picture of the rock before your inner eye, the more the gloom and depression in you actually crumble away ... ... just as in your daydream ... ... exactly as in this daydream ... ... Let the wind continue to blow over the rock, because with each gust of your breath, something falls from the rock ... ... It crumbles, and small pieces fall off of it ... ... Sand trickles down, and the rock gets smaller ... ... Conscious and deliberate breathing leads to inner relaxation ... ... Inner relaxation leads to the dissolution of depressive thoughts and feelings ... ... and inner pictures create reality ... ... So imagine very clearly how the rock of depression becomes smaller before your inner eye because it is being worn away by the wind of your breath ... ... Like in a time-lapse, sand and small stones trickle off the rock of depression everywhere ... ... The rock gets smaller and smaller ... ... this happens before your inner eye and thus deep in your feeling ... ... Depression crumbles to dust ... ... Focus simply on the picture of the rock that is getting smaller ... ... Pay attention to feeling your breath clearly ... ... The more clearly you can feel your breath and follow its rhythm, the more the rock also dissolves and crumbles to dust ... ... The rock crumbles to dust and with it the significance it has in your daydream

… … Depression crumbles to dust … … Depression crumbles to dust … …

Your body takes this in … … Your whole organism remembers these pictures exactly … … a rock of depression … … the gust of your own breath … … The trickling of the sand grains on the rock … … the crumbling of the boulder … … the crumbling of your depressive thoughts and feelings … … and thus creates space for new strength and confidence … … Every focus on your breathing, every attention to the flow of your breath reminds your organism to continue wearing down this rock and making it smaller and smaller … … and thus creates space for new strength and confidence … … and thus creates space for new strength and confidence … …

#6

Negative thoughts are not immutable... ... Depression is not simply there... ... Perhaps you have heard that depressive traits or low moods are already ingrained in the personality... ... But in our personality and even in our genes, there are infinite possibilities and opportunities... ... Every person can have positive and constructive thoughts... ... so can you... ... You had them before too... ... Just think back to an earlier time, a time when you mostly had very positive thoughts... ... Back then you were often cheerful and carefree... ... You could be happy and have fun... ... Then again, there were also bad events or worries that brought you down... ... But not for such a long time, because actually, our mood goes up and down... ... sometimes we are happy, then again sad... ... depending on what is happening... ... But at some point, this change was lost... ... Your mood just stayed depressed, even when beautiful events happened... ... So you want to come back... ... back to this change in mood so that the depressed mood dissolves... ... In your childhood, your mood was constantly changing with the events and experiences around you... ... That's normal, that's good... ... and it can be like that again, maybe even today... ... or a bit more every day... ... You know this also from adulthood... ... even then there was a time when everything was still the way it was in childhood... ... when moods were still appropriate reactions to events and experiences... ... But over time it happened that the melancholic thoughts were there more and more often... ... The more you then thought about the connections that made you sad or depressed, the clearer was this feeling of depression and hopelessness... ... when you were distracted or, more precisely, focused on other contents or things, different feelings were quickly in the foreground... ... and always when you understood what made you sad or depressed, when you worked through and resolved the backgrounds, the feelings also went away... ... It can be the same with your current depression... ... if you understand or let go of what makes it so clear and big in your perception, the depression will also become smaller... ... You can now start to let go of many things that make you so attentive to the bad mood and thus make the depressive thoughts smaller, maybe even dissolve or end them soon... ... because your whole organism will react to the inner changes, to your letting go... ... So now focus on your head and imagine all the thoughts in your head as small beads in different colors... ... There are red beads for all fear thoughts... ... You have often had fears and worries... ... Fear has also influenced your mood... ... sometimes even the idea of losing the depression can be frightening... ... Part of the depression may have already become routine, keeping you from changing and clarifying other difficulties because the negative thoughts are so much in the foreground... ... If you let go of fear, you can also let go of this part of fear and thus depressive thoughts... ... So you exhale the red fear thoughts with the next breaths... ... Imagine blowing up a balloon with each exhale and blowing your fear thoughts into this balloon... ... With every breath, you blow up the red balloon of fear more and let go of these fear thoughts... ... The fear thoughts are only in the red balloon now... ... The balloon eventually rises and slowly floats up to the sky... ... It is as light as a gas balloon and with the lightness of the balloon that rises higher and higher and takes the fear thoughts with it, it becomes lighter in you... ... lighter and freer... ...

... ... Then there are the many worrying thoughts that keep circling... ... the constant brooding and pondering... ... like thoughts that force themselves on you and you can't easily switch off... ... You find these thoughts as small yellow beads in your head... ... In your imagination, in your vision, you can look into your head and find these yellow beads of brooding... ... You can also exhale these thoughts and now blow up a balloon... ... The balloon fills with your breath and at the same time with your yellow thoughts of brooding... ... With every breath, you blow up the yellow balloon of circling thoughts more and let go of the brooding... ... The circling thoughts are only in the yellow balloon now... ... The balloon eventually rises and slowly floats up to the sky... ... It is as light as a gas balloon and with the lightness of the balloon that rises higher and higher and takes the brooding with it, it becomes lighter in you... ... lighter and freer... ... You look up at the sky and see many red balloons with your fear thoughts and many yellow balloons with your brooding... ... They float higher and higher... ... towards the sky, to dissolve there forever... ... and with the rising of the balloons that fly higher and higher, it becomes lighter in you... ...

because you free yourself with this image of floating balloons from fear and from circling thoughts... ...

Your depression can indeed dissolve... ... You can always ensure that what has made your mood so melancholic in your perception and interpretation dissolves like a balloon floating up to the sky... ... Just like here and today, you can imagine every day in a time of conscious breathing that fear that has held your depression in place floats up in red balloons to the sky... ... that circling thoughts that could slow you down float up in yellow balloons to the sky... ... and depression floats up with them and dissolves... ... depression floats up with them and dissolves... ...

#7

Ideomotorics refers to the phenomenon that our body follows our feelings and thoughts with movements. In everyday life, this following shows as posture, muscle tension, and movement patterns of a person, which naturally change with the mood and thoughts. In trance, ideomotor signals can be used to obtain information that the client cannot actively communicate. The subconscious can, for example, answer questions with an agreed finger signal. Naturally, ideomotor reactions can also be used suggestively, for example, with arm levitations and catalepsy. The following application can be done without trance induction and therefore has even more impact. An ideomotor reaction (upward movement of the right arm and downward movement of the left arm) is generated to show the client that it is the images and ideas in their thoughts that create their truth of depressive thought patterns. This is intended to strengthen the belief in possibilities for change through new thoughts and new images. Of course, the whole thing can also be done after a thorough trance induction, but I *recommend avoiding this because it makes a greater impression. Experienced hypnotists know: ideomotorics also works without hypnosis, but when it works, it is hypnosis!*

You probably cannot simply read aloud the following text as you would with all the others. However, I encourage you to try this variant once. It does not depend on the formulations but on the procedure. You don't have to memorize every word.

Explain to your client now that they should stand with both arms stretched forward. The palm of the left hand should face up, and the palm of the right hand should face down. Then they should imagine a heavy object, a thick book, or a stone on the left hand. At the same time, they should imagine a gas-filled balloon tied with a string to the right wrist. Then suggest that the heavy object is pressing the left hand down, and the gas balloon is pulling the right hand up. Repeat the suggestion a few times. Very quickly, the left arm will move down, and the right arm will move up. The client will simultaneously feel that the left arm actually becomes heavier and the right lighter. This is a simple exercise sometimes done as a suggestibility test. It always works, even if a client tries to resist the effect. They will feel it, and their arms will visibly react. The whole thing can run with a very wide scissor movement of the arms or with "only" ten centimeters distance. But that is enough. Clients are impressed by the exercise even if they already know it. And it still works. Just try it yourself without suggestion to see what happens when you stretch your arms forward as described and imagine both images, heavy stone and gas balloon, intensely with closed eyes. You will see: Your arms react to it!

You don't need a text template since you don't have to read this simple exercise. Nevertheless, I have written a short text example here as a guideline. I often do the exercise in courses and prefer to work standing. But it also works sitting or lying on a narrow couch.

Text Guide as Orientation:

... ... Stand upright, stable on both legs. And now stretch your arms forward. Very relaxed, not overextending. Good. Now turn the palm of your left hand upwards so that you could place something on it. And the right hand faces down. Good, let's start … …

… … Close your eyes and keep your arms like that … … Now imagine putting a very heavy stone on your left hand… … In your mind, place a heavy stone on your left hand and tie a gas-filled balloon to your right wrist… …

… … On the left hand lies a very heavy stone and the right hand is pulled up by the balloon… …

… … On the left hand lies a very heavy stone and the right hand is pulled up by the balloon… …

[Repeat the two images and observe the client's arms. You don't need a special trance tone in your voice. You can continue to speak "normally," perhaps even a bit faster than usual. Repeat the two images either always the same or with different words until the left arm slowly sinks down and the right arm moves upwards. This will happen very quickly. It is very simple and works for any layperson even without trance and without any knowledge of hypnosis, trance, or suggestion.]

… … Now keep your arms like this and open your eyes… … Look at your arms! … …

Let the client be amazed now. Most people are very surprised that it worked. Although the arm movement is usually felt even with closed eyes, many are unsure if it is a trick, if they are just imagining the movement. The more intense the surprise that the arms have actually moved and (mostly) so far apart. Discuss with the client again that it is only the thoughts and images in their head that create this truth. Just as it is only the images in their head that produce their depression. Conversely, this means, of course, that new images or new thoughts can also produce new attitudes.

This exercise is quite boring as a suggestibility test because no one needs such a test. As an introduction to therapy, however, the exercise can be very useful and helpful, for example, to show that images and ideas can indeed influence us very quickly and very clearly, against the knowledge of our mind. The mind knows that there is no object on the left hand and no balloon pulling on the right. Suggest to the client to repeat the exercise again to see and verify for themselves that the effect is still noticeable even when they know what will happen beforehand.

#8

You are here today to deal with your mood, especially the worries and fears that have weighed you down and dragged you down repeatedly... ... Everything that lies in our memory is also found in our body... ... everything that is deep in our soul is deep in our body... ... Every single thought, every mood... ... all our feelings manifest in our body... ... showing there as a physical sensation ... ... as pressure ... ... as tension ... ... as a strange feeling ... ... sometimes even as pain ... ... or just a strange tingling ... ... sometimes as a feeling of heaviness ... ... If you can clearly perceive your body, you can also achieve everything you have set out to do... ... recognize everything... ... and transform everything... ... let go of everything that has burdened you for too long, to be lighter and more cheerful again... ...

... ... Somewhere in your organism are also the worries and fears that have led to this depressed mood... ... There also sits this thought pattern that has repeatedly led to holding on to old worries and fears... ... Let's call it your depression pattern... ... It sits somewhere deep inside you and acts from there without you having noticed it... ... But now you know you don't need it anymore... ... You have long understood that there is this special pattern... ... You have accepted that it is there... ... At the same time, you have set out to find it and dissolve it... ... It is anchored in your feelings and thoughts, but also in your body... ... You can even feel it in your body, you can feel it... ... Maybe you know that you can feel everything that belongs to you physically if you come to rest, as you are now... ... and focus on your body... ... as you are now... ... Then you feel your depression as tension... ... or as warmth or cold... ... as pressure or in another way... ... All thought patterns that we carry deep within us show themselves most clearly at a specific spot in our body... ... as a signal that we can actually feel... ... So a signal of your depression shows itself in your body, which can warn you... ... so that you do not fall into the trap of brooding or grieving again... ... so that you can take better care of yourself... ... You just need to recognize this spot, then you can work on it and build a new pattern... ...

... ... Now direct your attention to your body and feel your body... ... Go from head to toe, as if you were standing next to yourself and could look at your body... ... and then find this special spot... ... Find this spot that feels somehow different because your depression pattern sits there... ... You find exactly the spot in your body where your depression has settled... ... Maybe you expected exactly this spot to catch your eye... ... or you are now occupying yourself in your perception with a spot on your body where you had not suspected the depression... ... But our feelings can show up everywhere... ...

You find the spot because it feels different... ... maybe just a little colder or warmer ... ... maybe as a tingling ... ... or as a slight goosebumps that suddenly forms ... ... Wherever this spot is ... ... There your depression pattern shows itself through a physical signal ... ... exactly there ... ... But even if you haven't found it yet ... ... It is there ... ... Then just take the spot that spontaneously comes to mind ... ... wherever that is ... ...

... ... Feel deeper and deeper into it ... ... Go entirely into this feeling ... ... whatever it may be ... ... It is your depression pattern that you feel there ... ... Maybe the spot feels completely different ... ... That is normal because many feelings are often side by side and confuse us ... ... But exactly at that spot, the depression sits in your body too … … Go deeper and deeper into this spot in your body and feel more clearly the signals of your body … … Maybe it feels strenuous or burdensome … … Maybe you thought that you had already overcome the depression more … … Don't worry, because here you mainly feel the thought pattern that has often led to your mood and thereby often to standstill … …

… … Now direct all your attention and all your mindfulness and loving care to exactly this point in your body and connect with the inner pattern that lies there … … Imagine how a small sun begins to shine from this spot … … Warm, pleasant sunlight flows from the small sun in your body and simply dissolves the old thought pattern … … The warm light of the sun in your body cleanses your entire organism … … dissolves the old thought pattern and creates new space for freedom and lightness … … All old patterns of fear and worry thoughts dissolve … … So more and more clarity arises deep within you … … This clarity can capture your entire body because you bring this mindfulness … … this attention to yourself … … More and more old entanglements dissolve and are replaced by new thought patterns of self-care and mindfulness ... ... Everywhere where the depression pattern was recently, you find more and more love from you for yourself ... ... more and more love from you for yourself ... ... your self-love and mindfulness ... ... your self-love and mindfulness ... ... Breathe calmly and evenly and trust in the strength within you ... ... Everywhere where the depression pattern was recently, you find more and more love from you for yourself ... ... more and more love from you for yourself ... ... your self-love and mindfulness ... ... your self-love and mindfulness ... ...

... ... You feel the change in your body and realize that your body can always show you how you are feeling ... ... especially in the feelings that you could not always feel so well in everyday life ... ... Now you can because you know that your body helps you ... ... So you pay attention to your body every day and ask yourself already in the morning when you get up how your body feels today ... ... It shows you when you need to take more care of yourself ...

#9

Depressive Brooding

Today you can embark on a special journey... ... a journey that takes you deep into your own creativity and imagination... ... The destination of this journey is always yourself... ... whatever you can and will experience always leads you back to yourself in the end... ... Your body shows you the way there... ... Just follow the rhythm of your breath and feel how it leaves your body with each exhale... ... Imagine that with the wind of your breath you could leave your body to embark on this journey... ... This journey that takes you away from the limitations of space and time... ... yet you always remain firmly connected to yourself and my voice... ... You are now leaving your body and entering the land of dreams... ...

You know these thoughts that circle so often and hardly let you go... ... It is sometimes as if they impose themselves... ... Then you take the thought and keep thinking... ... see all thoughts so worried... ... Again and again, you have tried to switch off these thoughts as well...

... But letting go of the thoughts was not always so easy... ... But that is exactly what you want to do today... ... Let go of thoughts... ... You want to finally have your peace and put your worries aside... ... Today it should and can be exactly like that... ... Today you let go of your thoughts... ... You simply let them go... ... because you want to and because now the time for freedom has truly come... ... Your thoughts are like letters you keep reading, they repeat and remain the same... ... You have read these thought letters all before and can no longer gain new insight from them... ... Your realization today is therefore to finally let go of these thought letters... ...

... ... You are outside in nature on a meadow... ... The weather is beautiful and you want to relax here in nature... ... find your peace... ... above all a nice peace of mind... ... That's what it's about today... ... peace of mind... ... You breathe in deeply and out, to inhale the fresh wind of nature and feel really free when you exhale... ... Then you take a few steps and hear the splashing of water... ... You let your gaze wander and see a small river flowing across the meadow... ... You walk towards the river and notice that you are carrying many letters in your hands... ... like a postman who forgot to deliver the letters where they belong... ... All these letters contain your recurring thoughts... ... Your thoughts that were always the same, that you have thought so often... ... You don't need these letters anymore because you already know their content... ... You already know what they say... ... You can no longer gain new insight, except for the insight that you can now let go of these thought letters... ... now you must let go... ... to feel free again and find peace... ... You already know everything you need to know... ... Letting go of these old thoughts is what it's all about now... ... By letting

go, you become free for truly new things... ... for new thoughts and ideas that you briefly consider, only to move on to the next thoughts and ideas... ... Then you see many bottles floating in the water of the river, they are sealed with corks and look like message bottles... ... But all the bottles are empty... ... You reach for these bottles and take the bottles floating close to the shore out of the water... ... You collect many bottles and put one of your thought letters in each bottle and seal the bottle again with the cork... ... You put all the thought letters in bottles and seal them until no thought is left... ... All circling thoughts you seal in the bottles… … Then you get ready… … ready to finally let go of the thoughts now… … It is time… … You let go of the thoughts today… … right now… … Then you throw the bottles with your thoughts into the river and watch them float away… … Maybe someone will read these thoughts someday, but you free yourself from them today because you already know them… … Your thoughts have long since fulfilled their purpose… … You have learned everything you could and had to from them… … Now you pass your thoughts on… … Now you give up your thoughts… … You say goodbye to exactly these thoughts that you know so well… … You let them go forever… … They remain as a memory, but now you let them go… …

You no longer need these thoughts… … You need new thoughts and new ideas… … new plans that come and go… … You firmly resolve to look at each new thought and then let it go again, because you quickly learn what is good for you and what you really need… … You really need peace and serenity… … peace and relaxation… … peace and freedom… … You watch the bottles drifting away and rejoice that they are already far away and floating further away with each second... ... You feel free and calm and prepare to remain free and calm... ... free and calm... ...

Then you lie down on the riverbank and just rest... ... You give yourself and your body peace and mindfulness... ... You consider that you can send disturbing thoughts on their way as message bottles every day... ... every day of your life you can be in the land of dreams by allowing yourself a moment of peace, closing your eyes and letting go of the message bottles of your thoughts in your imagination... ... Imagination and reality are very close together and in the land of dreams, both are the same... ... Then you think about how the land of dreams is deep within you... ... It has always been there... ... I'm just telling you about it...

#10

Feelings of Guilt and Self-Accusation

In our nightly dreams, everything is possible that we can imagine... ... there are no limits, we do not need logic and reason... ... Our feelings create the inner images and scenes that can help us learn more about ourselves... ... understand more about ourselves... ... be closer to ourselves... ... In our daydreams, it is exactly the same... ... they also have no limits... ... Daydreams also allow us the same insight into our deep inner self... ... into the realm of the unconscious and feelings... ... It is always our feelings that create our dreams... ... You find every single dream in this special land within you... ... in the land of dreams... ... Your breath carries you there... ... It blows your thoughts like a gentle wind into the land of dreams... ... Now... ...

You are standing on the field of insight, where you can discover so much... ... more than you could ever learn about yourself in your thoughts... ... So much about yourself... ... And with full confidence, you walk right through the field... ... It looks as if the whole field moves like a gentle wave in the wind... ... and with the feeling of the gentle wave movement, you relax deeper and deeper... ... You discover three huge crystal balls lying in the middle of the field of insight... ... They are so large that you can go inside... ... You approach the first ball... ... It is the ball of past people... ... All the people in your past who contributed to your feelings of guilt and thus your negative thoughts, you can meet here... ... Perhaps you know that all relationships we have somehow contribute to our life, sometimes helpful and good, and sometimes they also contribute to difficulties without us noticing... ... You know your bad conscience, which also shows itself when you have no omissions... ... But again and again, you think you have not done enough... ... have failed in life... ... This thought then gnaws at you and your mood gets worse and worse... ... But today it is time to let go of these guilt thoughts because you are innocent... ... really innocent... ... You go into this ball and look around... ... And gradually, all the people in your life appear... ... And those who contributed most to your bad conscience come closer... ... You see them more and more clearly... ... Maybe you expected some, others might surprise you... ... Maybe there are many people in this ball, maybe just a few or only one...

... Back then, you learned to take on the guilt that was not your own... ... learned to have a bad conscience... ... But today it is different... ... Today you are here to learn from the same people how to let go of these old guilt thoughts now because they belong to the past... ... You learn it from them now... ... Then you say goodbye to the people or the one and go outside onto the field of insight. You leave the people in the past because that is where they belong... ...

You continue walking and come to another ball. It is the ball of past situations... ... All situations, all events in your life that contributed to these guilt thoughts becoming so strong, these feelings of guilt appearing so quickly, are in this ball... ... You go inside, and the ball is empty... ... But gradually the important events show themselves... ... Whatever you can recognize in this ball... ... And even if you see nothing and no thought comes to mind - you can trust that all the events of your life are here... ... They work deep within you and help you learn something new today... ... Once you learned to take on guilt... ... Today it should be different... ... Today you learn from the same events, from the same situations and occurrences how to carry only the responsibility that truly belongs to you... ... Then you say goodbye to the situations.

You give them to the past because that is where they belong... ... You go outside again and walk further through the field... ...

You come to a third ball. It is the ball of your feelings... ... All your feelings are here in this ball... ... You go inside... ... There are also beautiful feelings here... ... Maybe you feel a special feeling... ... one that you haven't felt for a long time... ... maybe you feel right now that there is much more than just heavy thoughts, that there is also lightness or confidence... ... or another feeling that you can feel so clearly right now... ... Maybe you see colors or shapes that represent your feelings... ... They are here, all your feelings, and especially the feelings that contribute most to the guilt thoughts fading even faster... ... Now you can let all that work in peace and calm... ... peaceful and calm... ... Today it is possible... ... Today it is exactly possible... ... Today you are here to benefit from your own feelings... ... You learn how to let go of guilt thoughts and the bad conscience... ... develop constructive thoughts and continue to learn how to free yourself from heavy thoughts... ... live with a good conscience... ... free from guilt thoughts... ... peaceful and calm... ... You say goodbye to the old feelings... ... to the old guilt that was never real... ... You no longer need it... ... Once the old feelings were so important, and even today you could learn from them ... Now you give them to the past, because that is where they belong, only there... ... You go out of the ball and go to the edge of the field... ... You find the great gate of inner freedom... ... It only shows itself when the time is ready to finally go through it and be free... ... and exactly this time has come today... ... The gate opens by itself as you approach... ... And with a big step, you go through it and are free... ...

You feel the feeling of freedom deep within you... ... and your mood gradually becomes happier and more relaxed... ... Here in the land of dreams, everything is possible, including your liberation forever... ... Then you think about how the land of dreams is deep within you ... ... It has always been there ... ... I'm just telling you about it...

Distribution, publication, and copying in any form are prohibited and subject to damages.

Overview of All Titles in the Series "Ten Hypnoses"

Volume 1: Smoking Cessation
Volume 2: Anxiety and Restlessness
Volume 3: Burnout
Volume 4: Reducing Overweight
Volume 5: Coping with the Past
Volume 6: Suicidal Thoughts and Attempts
Volume 7: Psycho-Oncology
Volume 8: Obsessions and Tics
Volume 9: Self-Confidence and Decision-Making
Volume 10: Grief Work
Volume 11: Psychosomatics
Volume 12: Chronic Pain
Volume 13: Depressive Thoughts
Volume 14: Panic Attacks
Volume 15: Domestic Violence, Victim Support
Volume 16: Post-Traumatic Stress
Volume 17: Exam Anxiety and Stage Fright
Volume 18: Anti-Violence Training, Offender Support
Volume 19: Addiction Tendencies
Volume 20: Social Phobia and Fear of Contact
Volume 21: Nail Biting
Volume 22: Self-Awareness and Self-Love
Volume 23: Teeth Grinding and Night Clenching
Volume 24: Feelings of Guilt
Volume 25: Fear in Crowds
Volume 26: Fear of Flying, Aviophobia
Volume 27: Fear in Enclosed Spaces, Claustrophobia
Volume 28: Tinnitus, Ear Noises
Volume 29: Fear of Heights
Volume 30: Neurodermatitis

Copying, publishing, and sharing with third parties are only permitted with the written consent of the author. Please observe the notes on copyright and usage.

Volume 31: Finding Inner Balance
Volume 32: Overcoming Loneliness
Volume 33: Fear of Illness, Hypochondria
Volume 34: Anticipatory Anxiety, Fear of Fear
Volume 35: Jealousy in Relationships
Volume 36: Driving Anxiety
Volume 37: New Start after Separation
Volume 38: Fear of Injections
Volume 39: Heart Anxiety Neurosis
Volume 40: Overcoming Resentment and Anger
Volume 41: Resolving Blockages and Positive Thinking
Volume 42: Stress Reduction, Stress Management
Volume 43: Body Relaxation
Volume 44: Deep Relaxation
Volume 45: Fear of the Dark
Volume 46: Falling Asleep and Staying Asleep
Volume 47: Compulsive Buying
Volume 48: Restless Legs Syndrome
Volume 49: Bulimia
Volume 50: Anorexia
Volume 51: Overcoming Nightmares
Volume 52: Imagined Deformity
Volume 53: Overcoming Distrust, Finding Trust
Volume 54: Processing Failures
Volume 55: Humiliation, Emotional Hurt
Volume 56: Distressing Compassion, Vicarious Suffering
Volume 57: Self-Forgiveness
Volume 58: Self-Awareness, Self-Confidence
Volume 59: Saying No
Volume 60: Assertiveness
Volume 61: Setting Boundaries and Self-Assertion
Volume 62: Decision-Making Ability

Volume 63: Success Orientation
Volume 64: Ruminating, Circular Thinking
Volume 65: Accepting Pregnancy
Volume 66: Birth Preparation
Volume 67: Spiritual Opening
Volume 68: Joy of Life and Inner Lightness
Volume 69: Patience and Inner Peace
Volume 70: Fibromyalgia and Rheumatism
Volume 71: Irritable Bowel Syndrome, Crohn's Disease
Volume 72: Fear of Nausea, Emetophobia
Volume 73: Stuttering and Cluttering, Speech Flow Disorders
Volume 74: Concentration and Knowledge Anchoring
Volume 75: Vitality and Spontaneity
Volume 76: Searching for Meaning and Finding Goals
Volume 77: Life Crises, Life Events
Volume 78: Workaholism, Goal Obsession
Volume 79: Helper Syndrome, Helpless Helpers
Volume 80: Medication Abuse
Volume 81: Gambling Addiction
Volume 82: Internet Addiction, Smartphone Addiction
Volume 83: Hoarding Disorder, Compulsive Collecting
Volume 84: Conspiracy Thoughts, Overvalued Ideas
Volume 85: Fear of Operations and Treatments
Volume 86: Fear of Aging
Volume 87: Travel Anxiety
Volume 88: Anxiety When Urinating, Paruresis
Volume 89: Fear of Intimacy and Togetherness
Volume 90: Fear of Blushing
Volume 91: Coming Out in Homosexuality
Volume 92: Charisma Training
Volume 93: Migraines and Chronic Headaches
Volume 94: Overcoming Allergies, Bronchial Asthma

Volume 95: Normalizing Blood Pressure
Volume 96: Compulsive Perfectionism
Volume 97: Sports Hypnosis, Motivation
Volume 98: Sports Hypnosis, Performance Enhancement
Volume 99: Determination and Focus
Volume 100: Encountering the Inner Child
Volume 101: Cravings, Binge Eating
Volume 102: Stimulating Metabolism
Volume 103: Bipolar Mood Swings
Volume 104: Borderline, Identity Crises
Volume 105: Hypomania, Euphoria, Mania
Volume 106: Restlessness, Agitation
Volume 107: Nervous Breakdown
Volume 108: Adjustment Disorders
Volume 109: Self-Alienation, Depersonalization
Volume 110: Ending Self-Pity
Volume 111: Primary Gain of Illness
Volume 112: Secondary Gain of Illness
Volume 113: Bullying, Victim Support
Volume 114: Letting Go of Envy and Jealousy
Volume 115: Fear of Spiders, Arachnophobia
Volume 116: Fear of Dogs or Cats
Volume 117: Fear of Strangers, Xenophobia
Volume 118: Excessive Worries, Generalized Anxiety
Volume 119: Strengthening Sense of Responsibility
Volume 120: Unrequited Love, Heartache
Volume 121: Work-Life Balance
Volume 122: Letting Go of Unattainable Goals
Volume 123: Allowing and Accepting Help
Volume 124: Letting Go of Adult Children
Volume 125: Tourette Syndrome
Volume 126: Life Changes and New Starts

Volume 127: Accepting Life in a Wheelchair
Volume 128: Understanding and Overcoming Homesickness
Volume 129: Understanding and Overcoming Wanderlust
Volume 130: Dizziness, Meniere's Disease
Volume 131: Overcoming Aggression
Volume 132: Cutting and Self-Harm
Volume 133: Hair Pulling, Trichotillomania
Volume 134: Postpartum Depression
Volume 135: For Relatives of Dementia Patients
Volume 136: Self-Harm, Artificial Disorders
Volume 137: Activating Self-Healing Powers
Volume 138: Preventing Depression Relapse
Volume 139: Reactive Psychoses, Follow-Up
Volume 140: Obsessive Thoughts and Impulses
Volume 141: Compulsive Checking
Volume 142: Compulsive Counting, Symmetry Obsession
Volume 143: Compulsive Washing, Cleanliness Obsession
Volume 144: Compulsive Questioning
Volume 145: Dissociative Paralysis
Volume 146: Phantom Pain
Volume 147: Overcoming Complaining
Volume 148: Hay Fever, Pollen Allergy
Volume 149: Sexual Abuse, Victim Support
Volume 150: Standing Strong Against Sexism, #metoo
Volume 151: Binge Eating
Volume 152: Overcoming Thoughts of Revenge
Volume 153: Detachment from the Aggressor, Stockholm Syndrome
Volume 154: Courage to Separate
Volume 155: Chronic Fatigue, Exhaustion
Volume 156: Fear of the Future, Existential Anxiety
Volume 157: Excessive Worry About Children
Volume 158: Fear of Failure

Volume 159: Ending Distrust and Control
Volume 160: Dejection, Dysphoria
Volume 161: Boreout, Chronic Boredom
Volume 162: Bipolar Disorders, Relapse Prevention
Volume 163: Mania, Relapse Prevention
Volume 164: Nihilism, Feelings of Worthlessness
Volume 165: Thumb Sucking
Volume 166: Being Brave
Volume 167: Being Proud
Volume 168: Overcoming Shyness
Volume 169: Being Able to Delegate Responsibility
Volume 170: Being Able to Show Emotions
Volume 171: Letting Go of Guilt, Victim Support
Volume 172: Processing Guilt, Offender Support
Volume 173: Mood Swings, Cyclothymia
Volume 174: Lack of Drive, Vital Sadness
Volume 175: Hearing Voices with Reality Reference
Volume 176: Confident Communication
Volume 177: Standing Up for Oneself
Volume 178: Taking New Paths
Volume 179: Confident Job Application
Volume 180: No Longer Being Taken Advantage Of
Volume 181: End of Submissiveness
Volume 182: Depressive Numbness
Volume 183: Mood Drops, Affective Incontinence
Volume 184: Mood Instability
Volume 185: Somatoform Disorders
Volume 186: Stomach Ulcer, Psychosomatic
Volume 187: Accepting Amputation
Volume 188: Overcoming and Letting Go of Hatred
Volume 189: Ending Accusations
Volume 190: Allowing Tears, Being Able to Cry

Volume 191: Finding and Sorting Repressed Feelings
Volume 192: Somatoform Pain
Volume 193: Living Autonomously
Volume 194: Anhedonia, Joylessness
Volume 195: Persistent Sadness
Volume 196: Obesity, Food Addiction
Volume 197: Parents of Abused Children
Volume 198: Letting Go and Letting Be
Volume 199: Childhood Sexual Abuse
Volume 200: Fear of Loss

www.ingramcontent.com/pod-product-compliance
Lightning Source LLC
Chambersburg PA
CBHW030459220526
45464CB00006B/2576